RETIRE WITH PURPOSE

A Guide to Making the Most of Your Golden Years

Lisa Rosewood

Table of contents

Hobbies

Painting

Music

writing

Baking and making food:

DIY projects and home improvement

Collecting and memorabilia

Outdoor Activities

Climbing and Nature Strolls

Landscaping and gardening

Sports

Water-based Exercises

Travel

Domestic travel destinations

International travel locations

Budget-friendly travel tips

Options for group travel

Volunteer Work

Opportunities for community service

Giving back

Inter-generational volunteerism

Socializing

Building and maintaining friendships

Club and group membership

Socializing online:

Learning

Taking Classes and Workshops

Pursuing educational interests

Online learning options

Conclusion

Introduction

An opportunity to begin on an exciting and

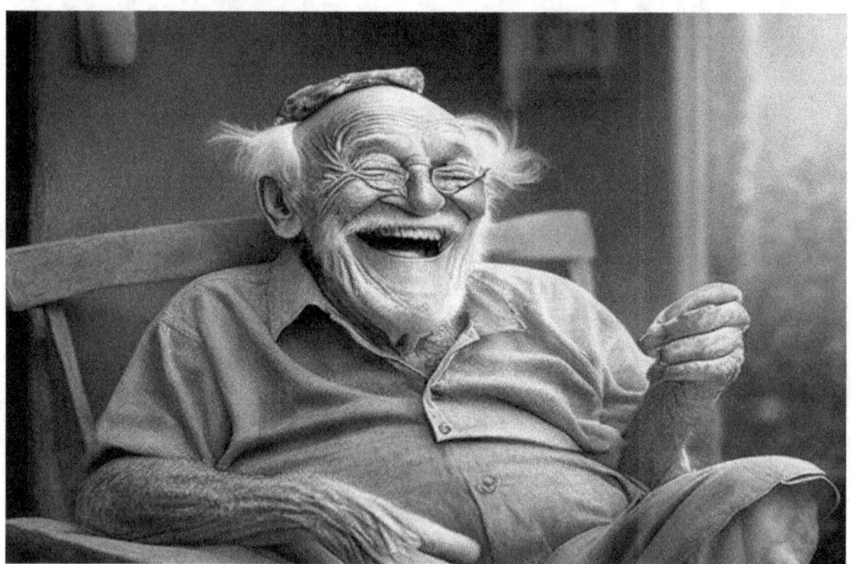

adventurous trip is retirement. Retirees now

have the option to pursue their unique hobbies

and take in their surroundings after years of hard

labor. Without the restraints of job or family

obligations, it's a time when you can concentrate

on what you want to achieve.

We'll look at a variety of activities that can make retirement a truly joyful and fulfilling period in this book. There is so much to look forward to, including going outside and experiencing nature, discovering new interests, traveling, giving back to the community, networking, and continuing to learn and grow.

With helpful suggestions and guidance on how to locate the activities that are ideal for you, we want to help you get started.

Hobbies

Retirement is the ideal chance to seek after your leisure activities and interests. Hobbies are activities you enjoy doing in your spare time without feeling obligated to produce a particular result or accomplish a particular objective. Hobbies can give you a sense of purpose and fulfillment, relieve stress, and improve your mental health.

For retirees who want to explore their artistic side and engage their minds in meaningful ways, creative pursuits like painting, writing, and music are excellent hobbies. There are a variety of ways to get involved in these creative activities and experience the joy and fulfillment they can bring, whether you're a seasoned pro or a novice.

Painting

People of all ages and skill levels can enjoy painting as a wonderful hobby. It's a great way to relax, unwind, and express your creativity while also producing something beautiful to share with others. To keep their minds active and creative juices flowing, retirees can paint ten different things:

Wild life: Wildlife is a popular subject for artists, whether it's a majestic eagle soaring through the air or a playful family of otters playing in the water. It is both challenging and rewarding to capture animals' natural beauty and essence in their natural environments.

The classic subject of painting is landscapes, which include peaceful lakes, majestic mountains, and rolling hills. From a bright and sunny day in the summer to a moody and misty morning in the fall, you can experiment with various techniques to create various moods and atmospheres.

Flowers and Plants: Flora is a popular and beautiful subject for artists, whether it's a colorful bouquet of flowers or a detailed painting of a single plant. You can create a vibrant and realistic image by experimenting with colors and textures.

Still Life: Painting everyday objects like books, vases, and fruits can be a challenging but enjoyable activity. Try different things with various lighting and points to make fascinating creations.

Portraits: Painting a portrait of a loved one can be a fun and intimate way to capture their essence and personality. Portraits are a great way to test your abilities, whether it's of a loved one, a pet, or a celebrity.

Abstract: If you want to try something new, abstract painting is a great way to let your creative juices flow. With no severe standards or rules, you can make an exceptional and beautiful magnum opus.

Seascapes - The sea and ocean side are generally a well-known subject for painters. Seascapes are a great way to show the power and beauty of the ocean, from waves crashing on the shore to a serene sunset over the water.

Cityscapes - The hurrying around of the city can be an extraordinary subject for painters. There is a plethora of options for constructing a one-of-a-kind and fascinating cityscape, from the bustling streets to the impressive skyscrapers.

Vehicles: Painting a variety of vehicles, from vintage automobiles to airplanes, can be both enjoyable and challenging. Catching the bends, subtleties, and shades of various sorts of vehicles can be an incredible method for testing your work of art abilities.

Abstract Realism is a great way to combine realism and abstract elements for those who want to push the creative envelope. By consolidating sensible subjects with dynamic strategies, you can make a novel and eye-discovering painting.

Music

Retirement is the ideal time to learn how to play an instrument, whether you have never played one before or want to get back into it. Start learning an instrument you like by taking lessons or by yourself using online resources.

Join an ensemble: If you enjoy singing, you might want to join a choir. It's a fun way to meet new people and get better at singing. Anyone, regardless of skill level, is welcome to join many choirs because there are no audition requirements.

Go to concerts: Attend live music performances and concerts when you have free time. This is an extraordinary method for finding new craftsmen and kinds, and to associate with other music fans.

Play with others: Joining a band or a group can be a pleasant method for playing music with others. Although there are numerous amateur groups out there that welcome new members of all skill levels, it can be a little intimidating at first.

Music you make yourself: Try your hand at writing your own music if you're feeling creative. To write lyrics or a simple melody, you don't have to be a musical genius.

Explore a variety of genres: Don't stick to just one kind of music. When you retire, it's a great time to try new music and listen to different kinds of music. Take a stab at paying attention to traditional music, jazz, blues, or world music.

Perform at music festivals: A great way to see multiple bands and artists in one place is at a music festival. Camping is a great way to combine your love of music with a short vacation because many festivals offer camping options.

Learn music hypothesis: Assuming that you're significant about your music side interest, think about learning some music hypothesis. You'll learn more about how music works and become a better musician and writer as a result.

Take part in charity events: To utilize your melodic abilities to reward your local area, think about playing for a noble cause occasion. Local musicians can perform at fundraisers and benefit concerts hosted by many organizations.

Use innovation to improve your music: There are a lot of apps and software programs out there that can help you write or play a musical instrument better. Take your love of music to the next level by leveraging technology to your advantage.

writing

For retirees who want to express themselves and explore their imaginations, writing is a great creative activity. Ten possible writing projects for retirees are as follows:

Individual journal: For your loved ones and

friends to enjoy, write your life story, capturing your memories and experiences.

Writing fiction: Let your imagination run wild as you create your own fictional world and characters.

Poetry: Try out a variety of poetry formats and explore the beauty of language.

Writing for trips: Write about the adventures and experiences you had while traveling to new locations.

Essays: Discuss a variety of topics, from personal philosophy to politics, with others.

Brief tales: Create short stories about a variety of topics and genres that can be read in one sitting.

Screenwriting: Compose a screenplay for a film or Television program, rejuvenating your story on the big screen.

Playwriting: Create a play for the stage that looks at the many different aspects of human experience and relationships.

Journalism: Spread the word about interesting stories or current events to a wider audience.

Blogging: Start a blog about something you're passionate about and connect with people who are interested in the same things as you.

Retirees can use writing as a therapeutic and fulfilling pastime to explore their creativity and share their thoughts and experiences with others. There is a writing project for everyone, whether you are interested in personal memoirs or fictional worlds.

Baking and making food:

Cooking and baking are two side interests that give delight as well as fill a viable need. Cooking your own meals is a great way to ensure that you are getting the nutrients your body needs as you get older. Maintaining a healthy diet is important as you get older.

Try out some new recipes: Trying out new recipes can be a fun and challenging way to improve your culinary skills. There is a plethora of recipes available online and in cookbooks. Think about trying new dishes, trying new ingredients, or making traditional dishes healthier by exploring new cuisines.

Cook for friends and family: Cooking can be a great way to spend time with loved ones and is frequently a social activity. Organize a cooking competition with friends or family or host a potluck where everyone brings a dish.

To begin a garden: Developing your own spices and vegetables isn't just a remunerating action yet can likewise give you knew and solid elements for your cooking. In the event that you don't have the space for a nursery, consider beginning a little spice garden on your windowsill.

Learn new cooking methods: Cooking techniques like sous vide and bread baking are among the most difficult to master. For new skills, think about taking a cooking class or watching tutorials online.

Bake for occasions special: Baking is a great way to celebrate birthdays, holidays, and other special occasions. Try out a new recipe for holiday cookies or make a cake or pie from scratch.

Try out a variety of baking techniques: There are a wide range of baking strategies, like involving a sluggish cooker or baking in a Dutch stove. Trying new approaches can be a fun way to test yourself and come up with new and delicious dishes.

Make your own preserves and jams: A fun and delicious way to use up extra berries or fruits is to make your own jams and preserves. Consider trying different things with various flavor blends or utilizing occasional fixings.

Take part in a cooking contest: Take part in a local cooking competition if you're feeling competitive. This can be a pleasant method for testing yourself and meet new individuals who share your adoration for cooking.

Make a cookbook for your family: A great way to pass on family recipes and customs to future generations is to create a family cookbook. Make a cookbook out of the recipes that members of your family have shared with you.

Go on a culinary journey: In the event that you love food, think about going on a culinary outing to investigate various cooking styles and culinary customs. Combining your passion for food preparation and travel can be a winning combination.

DIY projects and home improvement

Do-It-Yourself (DIY) undertakings and home improvement can be an incredible way for retired folks to remain dynamic and drew in while likewise working on their residing space. Whether you're a carefully prepared Do-It-Yourself lover or simply beginning, there are a lot of tasks that you can embrace to keep yourself occupied and enhance your home.

Home maintenance: You might find that as a retiree, you have more time to work on home improvements. Fixing dripping faucets, replacing light fixtures, or patching holes in the walls are all simple ways to improve the overall appearance of your home.

Refurbishing of furniture: On the off chance that you have a skill for working with your hands, consider renovating old furniture pieces. Refinishing, painting, or reupholstering an old piece of furniture can give it a new look. This is an extraordinary cash saving tip while likewise giving your home a one of a kind and customized touch.

Painting: Painting is another Do-It-Yourself project that can change the appearance of your home. Painting is a fun and satisfying project that you can complete on your own, whether it's a new color for your front door or a new coat of paint for the walls.

Landscaping: Not only is landscaping a great way to enhance the appearance of your home, but it can also provide exercise and fresh air. You can add blossom beds, plant trees, or make a vegetable nursery. By picking your own fresh produce, not only will it look great, but you will also be able to enjoy the results of your labor.

Carpentry: Take on a bigger project like building a bookshelf, birdhouse, or garden bench if you're handy with a saw and hammer. Although carpentry projects can be difficult, the end result is an attractive and useful addition to your home.

Energy-proficient redesigns: Not only can upgrading your home to be more energy efficient help the environment, but it can also help you save money on your monthly utility bills. You can put in new windows, add insulation, or buy new appliances that use less energy.

Automating your home: With the ascent of brilliant home innovation, you can robotize numerous parts of your home, including lighting, security, and temperature control. To make your home safer and more convenient, smart devices like doorbells, cameras, and thermostats can be installed.

Woodworking: Woodworking is a versatile pastime that can be used to build furniture as well as small decorative items. You can make beautiful and useful items for your home with the right tools and basic skills.

Plumbing: Although plumbing isn't the most glamorous DIY project, it can help you save money and feel like you accomplished something. Installing a new showerhead, replacing a toilet, or fixing a leaking faucet are all options.

Electrical work: You can tackle electrical projects like rewiring a room, adding outlets, and installing new light fixtures if you are comfortable working with electricity. Simply make certain to adhere to somewhere safe rules and counsel an electrical technician on the off chance that you're uncertain about any part of the undertaking.

Home improvement and DIY projects are great ways to keep busy and active in retirement. Besides the fact that they increase the value of your home, yet they likewise give a feeling of achievement and fulfillment. Keep in mind to begin with smaller tasks and progress to larger ones as you gain experience and confidence.

Collecting and memorabilia

Retirees can discover, learn about, and investigate the history and culture of various communities and nations through the engaging and fulfilling hobby of collecting and memorabilia. Gathering and memorabilia include the securing, show, and conservation of items that have authentic, social, or individual importance. Here are a few thoughts for retired folks keen on gathering and memorabilia:

Stamps: Stamp gathering is a well-known and captivating side interest that has been around for a really long time. Stamps from various nations, time periods, and themes, such as animals, sports, and history, can be collected by collectors. Stamp collecting can help retirees learn about art, geography, and history. It requires careful attention to detail, research, and patience.

Coins: Another well-liked pastime is coin collecting, which entails the acquisition and study of coins from various nations, periods, and materials. Coin collectors can learn about history, economics, and politics while collecting coins based on their rarity, historical significance, or beauty. In addition, accurate coin identification and evaluation necessitate expertise and research when collecting coins.

Antiques: Antiques are items with historical or cultural significance, beauty, and age. Furniture, artwork, pottery, glassware, and other items are examples of antiques. To identify, assess, and preserve antiques, collecting them necessitates expertise, knowledge, and research. Antique stores, flea markets, and online auctions all carry antiques.

Memorabilia: Memorabilia is a type of collecting in which items related to a specific event, person, or activity are acquired and displayed. Autographs, sports memorabilia, movie posters, and other items are examples of memorabilia.

Memorabilia collecting can help retirees connect with their favorite celebrities, athletes, or historical figures. It requires passion, research, and knowledge of the subject.

Art: Craftsmanship gathering is a side interest that includes the obtaining and enthusiasm for workmanship from various periods, styles, and specialists. Paintings, sculptures, prints, and other artifacts can be collected by art enthusiasts for their artistic value, beauty, or historical significance. Identifying, evaluating, and preserving art requires expertise, taste, and knowledge.

Books: The hobby of book collecting entails the acquisition and appreciation of books from a variety of genres, eras, and authors. First editions, signed copies, rare books, and books about their interests or hobbies are all options for book collectors. To identify, evaluate, and preserve books, book collecting requires expertise, knowledge, and research.

Music: Music collecting is a pastime in which one acquires and appreciates music from various periods, genres, and artists. Based on their rarity, sound quality, or historical significance, music enthusiasts can collect digital music, vinyl records, CDs, or cassettes. To identify, evaluate, and preserve music, music collecting necessitates expertise, taste, and knowledge.

Gathering and memorabilia is a side interest that can give retired folks a feeling of motivation, achievement, and satisfaction. It has the potential to assist retirees in developing new abilities, discovering new interests, and connecting with other collectors and enthusiasts. In addition to discipline, patience, and research, collecting memorabilia can keep retirees mentally and physically active.

Outdoor Activities

Activities in the Great Outdoors In your retirement, there are a lot of things you can do to get outside and enjoy nature. Here are ideas to start with

Climbing and Nature Strolls

Climbing is a fabulous method for investigating the outside and remain dynamic. Whether you're searching for a comfortable walk or a difficult journey, there are trails to suit each degree of capacity. When planning your hike, consider the following additional subpoints:

Choosing an appropriate trail: When choosing a trail for your fitness level, take distance, terrain, and elevation gain into consideration.

Getting ready for your hike: Make sure you have the right gear, like water, snacks, and sturdy shoes. Also, it's a good idea to tell someone where you're going and when you expect to be back.

Taking in the view: Spend some time taking in the natural splendor that surrounds you. To record your journey's sights and sounds, bring a camera or sketchbook.

Nature strolls are one more incredible method for partaking in the outside. They offer a more loosened up pace than climbing, permitting you to take in the landscape at a relaxed speed. A few extra sub-focuses to consider while arranging your inclination walk include:

Choosing an area: Look for botanical gardens, parks, and nature preserves in your area that offer guided tours or walking trails.

Dressing suitably: Dress for the weather and put on shoes that are comfortable. As required, bring sunscreen, a hat, and insect repellent.

Noticing natural life: Watch out for birds, bugs, and different creatures. Bring a field guide with you to help you identify them.

Landscaping and gardening

Gardening is a well-liked pastime among retirees, and for good reason. It gives you a lot of advantages, like exercise, fresh air, and the satisfaction of seeing your hard work bear fruit in the form of pretty flowers or abundant crops.

When planning your landscaping or gardening projects, other subpoints to keep in mind include:

Picking the right plants: When choosing plants for your garden or landscape, consider factors like sun exposure, soil conditions, and climate.

Organizing your design: Think about variables like the size and state of your space, as well as any current designs, while arranging your nursery or scene plan.

Taking care of your garden: Your garden or landscape needs to be watered, pruned, and weeded on a regular basis to stay healthy and beautiful.

Sports

Sports is a popular activity among retirees and there are different types of sports that can keep you engaged and active in retirement. Think about choices like:

Tennis: Playing this sport indoors or outdoors gives you a great workout.

Swimming: Swimming is a full-body workout with low impact that is easy on the joints.

Biking: Whether you favor relaxed rides or seriously testing territory, trekking is an incredible method for getting outside and investigate your general surroundings.

Water-based Exercises

Water-based exercises like swimming, kayaking, and fishing offer an incredible method for remaining cool and dynamic throughout the mid-year months. When planning your water-based activities, other sub-points to keep in mind include:

Picking the right movement: When choosing a water-based activity, consider factors like your level of water confidence and ability to swim.

Getting ready for your event: Ensure you have the legitimate stuff, including a day to day existence coat, sunscreen, and water. Also, it's a good idea to tell someone where you're going and when you expect to be back.

Taking pleasure in the event: Take the time to take in the water's awe-inspiring beauty.

Travel

Retirement can be the ideal time to visit old favorites and discover new ones. Retirees can take advantage of the numerous travel opportunities that are available to them because they have the freedom to travel without having to worry about work schedules or other commitments. To get you started, here are some suggestions:

The United States of America's diverse cultures, landscapes, and tourist attractions can all be thoroughly enjoyed through domestic travel. With just enough examination and arranging, retired people can set out on essential undertakings, learn new things, and associate with the nearby networks. Consider the following

Domestic travel destinations

Wilderness areas: The US has 63 public stops that safeguard and safeguard the absolute most shocking normal marvels and natural life environments. From the famous Stupendous Ravine in Arizona to the lofty Yellowstone in Wyoming and Montana, retired folks can investigate nature, climb trails, camp, and notice untamed life.

Historic Towns: In its cities, the United States of America has a rich history and culture. Retirees can learn about the country's colonial past, civil war, and cultural heritage in Boston, Philadelphia, New Orleans, and Charleston. Retirees can take walking tours, visit museums, savor the local cuisine, and observe the distinctive architecture and customs.

Beach front Escapes: There are more than 12,000 miles of coastline in the United States, and retirees can take advantage of some of the most stunning beaches, scenic drives, and seaside towns. From the bright Florida Keys to the rough shore of Maine and the Pacific Northwest, retired people can unwind, swim, kayak, and absorb the sun.

National Memorials and Monuments: Over a hundred national monuments and memorials honor significant individuals, events, and places in the United States. Retired folks can visit destinations like Mount Rushmore, the Sculpture of Freedom, the Lincoln Dedication, and the

Alamo, and find out about the country's set of experiences and commitments.

Festivals of Art and Music: The music and arts scene in the United States is well-known, and retirees can attend festivals and events that highlight the best talents and genres. Retirees can enjoy live music, theater, film, and visual arts at a variety of events, including the New Orleans Jazz Fest, South by Southwest in Austin, and the Sundance Film Festival in Park City.

International travel locations

There are numerous international locations that retirees can explore, and international travel can be an exciting and enriching experience. Consider these international travel destinations:

Europe: Europe is a popular retirement destination due to its extensive history, numerous cultures, and picturesque landscapes. Beautiful architecture, world-class art museums, and delectable cuisine can be found in countries like Italy, France, Spain, Greece, and Portugal. The continent can also be explored on river cruises along the Danube, Seine, and Rhine.

Asia: Asia offers a different scope of movement encounters, from the clamoring roads of Tokyo and Hong Kong to the serene sanctuaries of Thailand and Bali. China, India, and Vietnam are additionally famous objections for retired folks looking for experience and social drenching.

South America: Peru's Machu Picchu, Ecuador's Galapagos Islands, and Argentina's Iguazu Falls are just a few of the stunning natural landscapes and vibrant cultures that can be found in South America. Chile, Argentina, and Brazil are likewise well-known objections for wine sampling and investigating nearby cooking.

Africa: Retirees can get a taste of the continent's many cultures, wildlife, and landscapes by traveling to Africa. South Africa, Tanzania, Kenya, and Morocco are famous objections for safari visits, while Egypt offers an opportunity to investigate old history and engineering.

New Zealand and Australia: The Great Barrier Reef and Milford Sound are among the stunning natural features found in these locations.

Retirees can take a road trip through the picturesque countryside or visit cities like Sydney and Melbourne.

While arranging worldwide travel, it's vital to consider factors like visa necessities, travel protection, and any important immunizations. To ensure a respectful and enjoyable trip, it's also a good idea to research the culture and customs of the area.

Budget-friendly travel tips

Traveling on a shoestring budget is a great way to see new places without breaking the bank. With a few preparation and examination, having a great time and important outing on a tight spending plan is conceivable. Traveling on a budget? Consider these suggestions:

Pick the best travel time: Travel when airfare, lodging, and tourist attractions are less expensive during off-peak seasons. Additionally, considering traveling on weekdays rather than weekends may result in lower costs.

Search for arrangements and limits: To be informed of exclusive discounts and offers, sign up for email alerts from travel websites, hotels, and airlines. Additionally, prior to booking, look for coupon codes and discounts.

Pre-book your trip: To take advantage of early booking discounts, make your reservations for tours, lodging, and flights in advance.

Additionally, this can assist you in securing the best deals and avoiding price hikes at the last minute.

Consider other accommodations: Hostels, vacation rentals, and homestays are all viable alternatives to expensive hotels. These choices can offer a more authentic travel experience and are frequently less expensive.

Utilize public transport: In addition to being a great way to learn about the culture of the area, public transportation is frequently less expensive than taxis or rental cars. Take into consideration traveling by bus, train, or subway.

Like a local, eat: Rather than eating at costly cafés, attempt road food or neighborhood markets. Not only is this frequently less expensive, but it can also be an excellent way to try local cuisine.

Organize your trip: Research free or cheap attractions and activities in advance. You might be able to save money and avoid spending money you don't need.

You can still have a great time exploring new places on a budget if you follow these suggestions.

Options for group travel

For retirees, group travel can be a fun and exciting way to see new places and make memories with others who share their interests. Here are some gathering venture out choices to consider:

Groups for senior travel: Many travel organizations offer gathering visits explicitly intended for seniors. Accommodations, transportation, meals, and activities are often included on these tours, which are led by knowledgeable guides who can explain the history and culture of the area.

Graduated class travel gatherings: Check to see if your college or university offers travel programs for alumni if you are a graduate. These projects frequently incorporate excursions to objections all over the planet and furnish chances to interface with individual alumni.

Travel groups based on religion: Consider joining a travel group based on your faith if you are religious. Trips to holy places and opportunities for spiritual development and reflection are provided by these groups.

Groups for adventure travel: Adventure travel groups offer trips like hiking, kayaking, and safari tours for retirees who want to travel in a more adventurous way. People who share a passion for the great outdoors and a sense of adventure frequently make up these groups.

Travel groups for volunteers: Consider joining a volunteer travel group if you want to help others while you travel. These organizations provide opportunities to participate in international community service projects while also learning about the local culture and attractions.

Volunteer Work

Volunteering can be a great way for retirees to stay active and involved while giving back to their community. Retirees have a variety of options for volunteering in the community, and they can choose to get involved in causes they are passionate about. Some examples of volunteer work for retirees include:

Opportunities for community service
Shelters and food pantries

Retirees can help those in need in a great way by volunteering at shelters and food banks. You can help with serving dinners, putting together food gifts, and figuring out garments and different things.

Animal sanctuaries: In the event that you love creatures, chipping in at a creature cover is an extraordinary choice for you. You can assist with dog walking and feeding, cage cleaning, and adoption events.

Mentorship and tutoring: Retirees can mentor or tutor younger members of their community by utilizing their expertise and skills. Helping someone achieve their goals and improve their skills can be a rewarding experience.

Conservation of Nature: Retired people can partake in charitable effort that spotlights on natural protection. Planting trees, cleaning parks and beaches, and promoting recycling are examples of activities.

Work as a Hospital Volunteer: Hospital patients and staff can benefit from volunteers' visits, meal delivery, and assistance with administrative tasks.

Retired people who are hoping to have an effect in their networks or past can track down various open doors for humanitarian effort. Not only does volunteering help the organization or cause being supported, but it also gives the volunteer a sense of purpose and fulfillment.

Giving back

Volunteer work is one-way retirees can help others and make a difference:

Support nearby foundations: Supporting local charities that assist those in need is one-way retirees can give back to their communities. This can be done by giving time or money to organizations that help people in need by providing food, shelter, medical care, and other services.

Tutor or mentor: Mentors and tutors can be retired individuals who are knowledgeable in a particular field or skill. This could mean working with adults who want to learn a new skill or trade or with students at schools or community centers.

Volunteer at nursing homes or hospitals: Volunteer opportunities can be found at nursing homes, clinics, or hospitals for retirees who have a passion for healthcare. Providing patients with companionship and emotional support, assisting with administrative tasks, or assisting with medical procedures are all examples of this.

Help with catastrophe alleviation: Volunteering with disaster relief organizations is a good option for retirees who want to make a difference during times of crisis. This can include assisting with clean-up and rebuilding efforts, providing supplies and shelter to disaster victims, or helping with search and rescue.

Support animals: Retired folks who have an affection for creatures can chip in at neighborhood creature covers, natural life communities, or zoos. Taking care of animals, assisting with medical procedures, or educating

the general public about animal welfare issues
are all examples of this.

Volunteerism among people of different
generations is known as inter-generational
volunteerism. In this type of volunteerism,
volunteers from different generations come
together to support a common cause. This type
of chipping in can be unimaginably gainful for
both more youthful and more established
people.

Inter-generational volunteerism

Intergenerational volunteerism can provide
seniors with a sense of purpose and fulfillment as

well as opportunities to share their expertise with younger generations. It can also combat feelings of loneliness or isolation and help seniors feel more connected to their communities.

Intergenerational volunteerism can provide younger people with valuable learning experiences and opportunities to acquire new skills. It can likewise assist them construct positive associations with more established grown-ups and gain a more noteworthy appreciation for the commitments of more seasoned ages.

Intergenerational volunteerism comes in many forms, from mentorship programs to community service projects. Some examples include:

Coaching or tutoring: Programs that match older adults with young people in need of academic support or mentorship are offered by numerous schools and community organizations. This could be as simple as helping a young person with their homework, offering advice on how to apply to college, or just being a positive adult presence in their life.

Art projects for all ages: When people of different generations come together to make something beautiful, collaborative art projects can be a fun and satisfying way to do so. This can incorporate exercises like composition paintings or making figures.

Chipping in at senior focuses: Numerous senior communities depend on volunteers to assist with exercises and occasions. Young volunteers can be of assistance in a variety of ways, including leading exercise classes, putting together games or other activities, or just spending time with older people.

Intergenerational administration projects: Service projects with older and younger volunteers can be a great way to unite different generations around a common goal. Volunteering at a food bank or cleaning up a neighborhood park are two examples of this.

Socializing

Retirement does not have to be a time of isolation or loneliness. In fact, it can be a chance to have fun, meet new people, and build meaningful relationships. Socializing is an important part of retirement that can make a big difference in one's life quality. In this part, we will investigate various ways of associating during retirement.

Building and maintaining friendships

Friendship is significant at any point in one's life, but it is particularly significant in retirement. A sense of belonging and purpose can be provided by strong friendships that support one another.

Keeping up with existing fellowships and fabricate new ones is fundamental. How to make and keep friends is as follows;

Take part in a group or club that interests you: A great way to meet new people with similar interests is to join a club or group centered on your interests. It provides an opportunity to socialize, exchange ideas, and learn new things.

Go to get-togethers: Participate in community gatherings like fairs, concerts, and other social events. It's an opportunity to socialize, have fun, and meet new people.

Volunteer: Volunteering in your community is a great way to help others and meet new people at the same time. A sense of purpose and belonging are provided by it.

Utilize tech: Keep in contact with loved ones who live far away utilizing online entertainment and video calls. It's a great way to stay in touch with their lives and build your relationship.

Club and group membership

During retirement, joining clubs and organizations is a great way to meet new people. A sense of belonging and a sense of purpose can be provided by clubs and groups based on common interests. Here are a few clubs and gatherings that retired folks can join:

Book groups: Book clubs are a great way to make new friends and talk about books.

Group workouts: Yoga, swimming, and walking are just a few of the activities that can be done in fitness groups to help people stay fit while also meeting new people.

Strict associations: A sense of community and belonging can be provided by religious organizations.

Participating in gatherings and events:

During retirement, going to events and gatherings is a great way to meet new people. It gives a chance to meet new individuals and have some good times. Retirees can attend the following events and gatherings:

Concerts: Concerts are a great way to enjoy music and meet new people.

Festivals: Socializing and having fun can be possible at festivals that focus on food, music, or other interests.

Events for sports: Games like football, b-ball, and ball games can give a chance to mingle and appreciate sports.

Socializing online:

Socializing online is a great way to stay in touch with distant relatives and friends. It gives them a chance to keep up with their lives, share information, and meet new people. Some online social activities include:

Media online: It is possible to keep in touch with friends and family via social media platforms like Instagram, Twitter, and Facebook.

Skype calls: Video calls utilizing stages, for example, Zoom and Skype give an amazing chance to have eye to eye discussions with loved ones who live far away.

Learning

The perfect time to learn new skills or pursue a passion you may not have had time for during your working years is when you enter retirement. There are many ways to keep your mind active and engaged in retirement, including taking a class, pursuing an educational interest, or even mentoring and tutoring others.

Taking Classes and Workshops

In retirement, taking classes and workshops is an excellent way to acquire new skills and maintain mental activity. Classes and workshops can take many forms, from formal university courses to informal community classes. Here are a few focuses to consider while chasing after this choice:

Personal passions: Choose workshops and classes based on your own interests. Assuming you're enthusiastic about a specific subject, like history, workmanship, or writing, search for classes that emphasis regarding that matter.

Continuing professional growth: Learning new skills for a part-time job or keeping up with changes in your field can be great goals for professional development in retirement. Find classes and workshops that will help you stay current in your field.

Neighborhood people group classes: Classes and workshops are available for a reasonable price at a lot of the community centers and adult education programs in the area. These classes, which can include cooking and language instruction, can be a fantastic way to meet new people in your community.

Online training: There are also a lot of online courses, many of which are free or cheap. Courses in a wide range of subjects are available on platforms like EdX, Udemy, and Coursera, which can be a convenient option for those who prefer to learn at home.

Programs for continuing education: There are a lot of universities and colleges that offer continuing education courses just for retirees. These projects can give admittance to college assets and offices, as well as an opportunity to draw in with other deep-rooted students.

Coaching and mentoring potential open doors:
You can also learn by becoming a mentor or tutor. You can learn from other people and share your expertise. Many schools and local area associations offer coaching and mentoring programs that give preparing and support.

Pursuing educational interests

Pursuing educational interests is a great way to keep your mind engaged and active. It can also be a satisfying way to learn about new things and investigate new subjects. Some things to think about:

Find out what you like to do: Think about the topics that interest you first. Is there a subject that has always intrigued you? Do you have any abilities you'd like to improve? Make a list of your interest areas.

Investigate educational options: Whenever you've recognized your inclinations, research instructive open doors that are accessible to you. Investigate online courses, universities, and community colleges in your area. Take into consideration taking part in a study abroad program, joining a book club or discussion group, or attending lectures or seminars.

Think about how you learn best: Different people learn differently. Some people like to learn through doing, while others like to read or

listen to lectures. Look for educational opportunities that cater to your preferred learning style.

Make use of free tools and resources: Podcasts, YouTube videos, and online courses are just a few of the many free educational resources available. Make use of these resources to gain knowledge about a wide range of subjects without spending a penny.

Maintain order: Maintaining organization is essential because pursuing educational interests can be overwhelming. Make a study plan and a list of the resources you'll need for each subject.

Get help from your friends: Think about joining a group of students who share your interests. This can be an extraordinary method for examining thoughts and offer information with other people who are chasing after instructive interests.

Be open-minded: Chasing after instructive interests can be testing, however keeping a receptive outlook is significant. Be open to learning about new subjects and considering different points of view. You'll be able to better comprehend the world around you as a result of this.

Online learning options

Options for Online Education Online education has grown in popularity recently, and for good reason. It offers an adaptable and helpful method for keeping on learning and investigating new themes, even in retirement. There are many options for online education, from free courses to more in-depth programs that might cost money. The following are some of the advantages and options of online education:

Flexibility: Flexibility is one of the biggest advantages of online education. From any location with an internet connection, you can access the course materials and complete assignments at your own pace. Whether you prefer to study in the morning, in the afternoon, or in the evening, this makes it simple to fit learning into your schedule.

A wide range of topics: A wide range of subjects, from history and literature to science and technology, can be accessed through online learning. Without the constraints of a conventional classroom setting, you can pursue your interests while also learning something new.

Free courses: Coursera, edX, and Khan Academy are just a few of the many platforms that provide free online courses. These courses can be short tutorials or more in-depth programs. They are a great way to learn about new subjects without having to commit to a long-term program.

Paid services: For the people who need to seek after more top to bottom realizing, there are likewise paid programs accessible. These programs can provide more structured and rigorous learning experiences and may be offered by universities or other educational establishments. Models incorporate Masterclass, Udemy, and Expertise share.

Courses with certificates: Certificate programs, which provide formal recognition of your completion of a course or program, are also offered by many online learning platforms. This can be a great way to show that you are knowledgeable and skilled in a particular field.

Interaction with others: Additionally, there are opportunities for social interaction with other students through online learning. You can share ideas and have meaningful conversations with other students and teachers by connecting with them through discussion forums and other platforms.

Opportunities for Mentoring and Tutoring
Mentoring and tutoring can be extremely

satisfying retirement activities. Besides the fact that they permit you to impart your insight and experience to other people, yet they likewise give a chance to have a beneficial outcome on somebody's life.

You can get involved in mentoring and tutoring in the following ways:

Help out as a volunteer at a school or community center: Volunteers are needed at a lot of schools and community centers to assist students with reading, writing, math, and science tutoring.

Take part in a mentoring program: For retirees, there are numerous mentoring programs, such as

Big Brothers Big Sisters, which matches adults with children in need of a positive role model.

Online, offer your services: Additionally, numerous online platforms, such as Tutor.com and Chegg, connect students with subject-specific tutors. You can work from home and set your own schedule thanks to these platforms.

Mentor a brand-new retiree: On the off chance that you have as of late resigned, consider turning into a tutor for somebody who is going to resign. You can share your experiences and offer guidance on how to make the most of retirement.

Become a sports team mentor or coach: Consider volunteering as a coach or mentor for a local youth sports team if you enjoy sports. Young athletes can benefit from your assistance in teaching them useful skills as well as your support and encouragement.

During retirement, mentoring and tutoring can be a great way to stay involved in your community and connected. Besides the fact that these exercises give a feeling of motivation and satisfaction, however they likewise permit you to have a beneficial outcome on the existences of others.

Conclusion

As we arrive at the finish of this book, it's memorably vital, the significance of remaining dynamic and connected with during retirement. Retirement can be a fun time filled with new opportunities for growth and exploration. By attempting new things and chasing after our inclinations, we can keep on tracking down significance and reason throughout everyday life.

Take the advice and information we've provided in this book and put it to use to plan a fulfilling retirement for yourself. Step outside of your comfort zone and try something new without hesitation. The options are endless, and they can include volunteering in your community, learning a new skill, or traveling to a new location.

Keep in mind, retirement is a valuable chance to make every moment count and partake in your rewards for all the hard work. Make the most of it, then! We hope that this book has inspired you and shown you how to do that in concrete ways.

There are numerous excellent books, websites, and organizations that can assist you in finding additional resources on how to maximize your retirement. We wish you all the best on your journey to retirement and encourage you to keep learning and exploring.

www.ingramcontent.com/pod-product-compliance
Lightning Source LLC
Chambersburg PA
CBHW051836250726
48659CB00005B/1877